Kidn
Cookbook (2021 Edition)

The Ultimate Cookbook for Improving Your Health, Burning Fat and Preventing Kidney Disease

Bianca Schneider

TABLE OF CONTENTS

INTRODUCTION

Low dietary protein levels slow the development of chronic kidney disease and decrease phosphorus - a hemodynamically mediated glomerular injury. Furthermore, a protein-restricted diet lowers the level of phosphorus in the body, which is linked to kidney progression and patient longevity. Calcium, iron, magnesium, potassium, and other nutrients all require phosphorus to be produced. Since phosphorus reaches the body by food and exits through the kidneys, it is extracted from the food, where it is thought to cause kidney damage.

Vegetarian kidney diets require a bespoke diet from a known nutritionist since vegetarian protein sources include differing levels of potassium and phosphorus. Since a kidney diet restricts nutrition, you must consume high-quality protein on a daily basis. The amount of protein you consume is determined by the severity of your kidney condition, so you can keep your body in good health. A protein-restricted diet must not reduce your levels. A high protein, low carbohydrate diet and never dehydration are the two most crucial things you can do to maintain kidney function from more deterioration.

Avoid beef: Cooked meat contains a lot of salt and protein, so it's best to eat it in moderation when it comes to kidney nutrition. In the short term, this can make people feel worse and undermine the effects of a kidney diet, but it can also lead to kidney failure.

Consult your veterinarian to find out which protein-rich drugs to stop and what recovery options are available. If CKD has advanced to IRIS (stage 3 CKD) or proteinuria has been detected, a commercial renal diet should be fed. If no azotemia is present, however, most patients will only be given the normal kidney diet for a limited duration if the procedure results in kidney failure.

Brown rice is rich in phosphorus and potassium, so it should probably be eaten in regulated and small amounts in kidney diets. To prevent high dietary intake of potassium or phosphorus, the easiest way to integrate brown rice into the kidney diet is to monitor portions and combine them with other ingredients.

People who are at a high risk of contracting kidney failure should have their kidney function tested and examined on a regular basis.

Kidney disease (kidney failure) is the disruption of natural kidney activity due to temporary or irreversible injury to the kidneys. Kidney failure, also known as the end stage of kidney disease, can occur at any time during the course of the disease.

Kidney function can deteriorate or worsen over time, resulting in kidney failure that can lead to complications such as kidney stones, kidney cancer, or the need for a kidney transplant. It's also known as developed renal failure (ERF), and it happens when almost all or all of a person's kidney function has been compromised, or the disease has become life-threatening. Medication, alternative medicine, nutrition, and lifestyle are also important aspects of diabetes care.

In the United States, chronic kidney disease is one of the most frequent forms of kidney failure. Improvements of chronic kidney disease (CKD) can be observed in as few as a few months or years.

People with kidney dysfunction, for example, have lower blood pressure and blood sugar levels than people who have normal kidney function. To prevent the buildup of such contaminants and nutrients in the blood, you must eat a kidney-friendly diet.

Royal Canin, a modern dry diet that combines hydrolyzed soy with low-phosphorus protein, has recently been launched and may be useful to people with kidney disease.

BREAKFAST

1. Buckwheat Pancakes

Preparation Time: 10 minutes

Cooking Time: 15 minutes

Servings: 4 servings

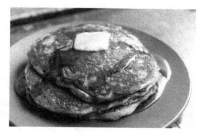

Ingredients:

- 1¾ cups homemade or unsweetened store-bought rice milk
- 2 teaspoons white vinegar
- 1 cup buckwheat flour
- ½ cup all-purpose flour
- 1 tablespoon sugar
- 1 large egg
- 2 teaspoons Phosphorus-Free baking powder
- 1 teaspoon vanilla extract
- 2 tablespoons butter, for the skillet

Directions:

1. combine the rice milk and vinegar. Let sit for 5 minutes.

2. Meanwhile, in a large bowl, mix the buckwheat flour and all-purpose flour. Add the sugar and baking powder, stirring to blend.

3. Add the egg and vanilla to the rice milk and stir to blend. Add the wet ingredients to the dry, and stir until just mixed.

4. melt 1½ teaspoons of butter. Use a ¼-cup measuring cup to scoop the batter into the skillet. Cook for 2 to 3 minutes, until small bubbles form on the surface of the pancakes. Flip and cook on the opposite side for 1 to 2 minutes.

5. Transfer the pancakes to a serving platter, and in batches, continue cooking the remaining batter in the skillet, adding more butter as needed.

Nutrition: Calories: 264; Total Fat: 9g; Saturated Fat: 3g; Cholesterol: 58mg; Carbohydrates: 39g; Fiber: 3g; Protein: 7g; Phosphorus: 147mg; Potassium: 399mg; Sodium: 232mg

2. Broccoli Basil Quiche

Preparation Time: 10 minutes

Cooking Time: 55 minutes

Servings: 8 servings

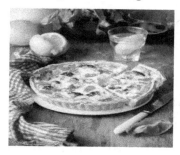

Ingredients:

- 1 store-bought frozen piecrust
- 2 cups finely chopped broccoli
- 1 tomato, chopped
- 2 scallions, chopped
- 3 eggs, beaten
- 2 tablespoons chopped basil
- 1 cup homemade rice milk or unsweetened store-bought rice milk
- ½ cup crumbled feta cheese
- 1 garlic clove, minced
- 1 tablespoon all-purpose flour
- Freshly ground black pepper

Directions:

1. Preheat the oven to 425°F.

2. Line a pie pan with the piecrust, and use a fork to pierce the crust in several places. Bake the crust for 10 minutes. Remove from the oven and reduce the temperature to 325°F.

3. In a medium bowl, mix the broccoli, tomato, scallions, eggs, basil, rice milk, feta, garlic, and flour. Season with pepper.

4. Pour the broccoli-and-egg mixture into the prepared pie pan. Bake for 35 to 45 minutes, until a knife inserted in the center comes out clean. Let cool for 10 to 15 minutes before serving.

Nutrition: Calories: 160; Total Fat: 10g; Saturated Fat: 3g; Cholesterol: 87mg; Carbohydrates: 13g; Fiber: 1g; Protein: 6g; Phosphorus: 101mg; Potassium: 173mg; Sodium: 259mg

3. Poor Knight with Apple Compote

Preparation Time 15minutes

Cooking Time: 0 minute

Serving: 4

Ingredients:

- 4 large (or 8 small) slices of white bread
- 80 ml of cream
- 120ml water
- 1 egg
- 1 teaspoon vanilla pudding powder (for cooking)
- 2 tbsp sugar
- Breadcrumbs
- 40g butter
- Sugar and cinnamon to taste
- 400g apple compote

Direction:

1. Mix the cream and water and stir together with the pudding powder, sugar, and egg until smooth. Halve or quarter the white bread slices and turn in the egg mixture.

2. Then turn in breadcrumbs and bake in hot butter over mild heat until golden brown on both sides.

3. Sprinkle with cinnamon sugar to taste and serve with the apple compote.

Nutrition: 416 calories 7g protein 192mg potassium 185mg sodium

4. Papaya and Cranberry Jam

Preparation Time: 8 minutes

Cooking Time: 10 minutes

Serving: 6

Ingredients:

- pulp of a ripe papaya 700 grams
- Lemon juice 4 tbsp
- Cranberries / Cranberries 100 grams
- Preserving sugar 1: 1 1000 grams

Direction:

1. With hot water, wash the papayas, rub them dry and peel them. Then cut it in half with a teaspoon and scrape the seeds out. With the lemon juice, purée the pulp. The cranberries are washed and sorted, put in a large saucepan, and lightly mashed with a fork. Add the papaya fruit puree and 1:1 of the gelling sugar and mix well.

2. While stirring, bring to the boil over high heat until all the food bubbles vigorously. Now the time for cooking begins! Let it simmer for 4 minutes, constantly stirring.

3. Remove the pot from the stove. Fill the hot mass quickly with jars rinsed with hot water to the brim and close immediately with the screw cap.

Nutrition: 344 calories 0.1g protein 31mg potassium 182mg sodium

5. Lemon Curd

Preparation Time: 5 minutes

Cooking Time: 75 minutes

Serving: 6

Ingredients:

- Freshly squeezed lemon juice 150 ml

- Freshly squeezed mango juice 100 ml

- Butter 100 gr.

- Sifted corn starch 30 gr.

- White wine dry 150 ml

- Sugar 150 gr.

- Grated lemon peel 1 pc.

Direction:

1. Melt the butter and heat the corn-starch while stirring until it is light yellow. Add lemon and mango juice and the white wine. Please make sure that there are no lumps.

2. Now add the sugar and lemon zest and let it cook for another 2 minutes. Fill everything into glasses immediately.

3. The lemon curd unfortunately only lasts about 3 days in the refrigerator.

Nutrition: 239 calories 0.3g protein 28mg potassium 171mg sodium

6. Pancakes with Raspberries and Ricotta

Preparation Time: 21 minutes

Cooking Time: 32 minutes

Serving: 2

Ingredients:

- 100g flour
- 1 egg
- 200 ml of mineral water
- 50ml cream
- 1 tsp baking soda
- 1 pinch of salt
- 2 tbsp rapeseed oil
- 80g raspberries
- 2 tbsp liquid honey
- 200g ricotta

Direction:

1. Mix the flour with the egg, mineral water, cream, salt, and baking powder.

2. Let the dough rest for 10 minutes and fry 2 pancakes in hot rapeseed oil.

3. Fill with ricotta and raspberries and pour the honey over them.

Nutrition: 574 calories 21g protein 294mg potassium 112mg sodium

7. Muesli Made from Rice Flakes

Preparation Time: 8 minutes

Cooking time 10 minutes

Serving: 2

Ingredients:

- 50 ml of cream
- 150 ml of water
- 2 tbsp sugar
- 35 g rice flakes
- 50 g blueberries from the glass, drained
- fresh mint

Direction:

1. Bring the cream and water to the boil in a saucepan, then add the rice flakes and sugar, bring to the boil again briefly and remove from the stove. Let it soak for 10 minutes.

2. Divide between 2 bowls, add blueberries, and serve with the mint.

Nutrition: 200 calories 2g protein 68mg potassium 10mg sodium

LUNCH

8. Beef Stir-Fry

Preparation Time: 5 minutes

Cooking Time: 15 minutes

Servings: 4

Ingredients:

- 4 cups water
- 2 tablespoons cornstarch
- 2 teaspoons honey
- 6 tablespoons Worcestershire sauce
- 1 tablespoon minced fresh ginger
- 1-pound boneless beef round steak, cut into thin strips
- 1 tablespoon olive oil
- 3 cups broccoli florets
- 2 carrots, thinly sliced
- 1 (6 ounce) package frozen pea pods, thawed
- 2 tablespoons chopped onion
- 1 (8 ounce) can sliced water chestnuts, untrained
- 1 cup cabbage
- ½ cup kale, chopped
- 1 tablespoon olive oil

Directions:

1. Combine corn-starch, honey, and Worcestershire sauce, in a small bowl until smooth. Stir in ginger; toss beef in sauce to coat.
2. Heat 1 tablespoon oil in a large skillet over medium-high heat. Cook and stir broccoli, carrots, pea pods, and onion for 1 minute. Stir in water chestnuts, cabbage, and kale; cover and simmer until vegetables are tender, about 4 minutes. Remove from skillet and keep warm.
3. In same skillet, heat 1 tablespoon oil over medium-high heat. Cook and stir beef until desired degree of doneness, about 2 minutes per side for medium. Return vegetables to skillet; cook and stir until heated through, about 3 minutes.

Nutrition: Calories 139, Total Fat 3.9g, Saturated Fat 0.8g, Cholesterol 12mg, Sodium 972mg, Total Carbohydrate 18.7g, Dietary Fiber 4g, Total Sugar 5.8g,

9. Vegetable Casserole

Preparation Time: 15 minutes

Cooking Time: 15 minutes

Servings: 8

Ingredients:

- 1 teaspoon olive oil
- 1 sweet onion, chopped
- 1 teaspoon garlic, minced
- 2 zucchinis, chopped
- 1 red bell pepper, diced
- 2 carrots, chopped
- 2 cups low-sodium vegetable stock
- 2 large Red bell peppers, chopped
- 2 cups broccoli florets
- 1 teaspoon ground coriander
- ½ teaspoon ground comminutes
- Black pepper

Directions:

1. Heat the olive oil into a big pan over medium-high heat.
2. Add onion and garlic. Softly cook for about 3 minutes until softened.
3. Include the zucchini, carrots, bell pepper and softly cook for 5-6 minutes.
4. Pour the vegetable stock, Red bell peppers, broccoli, coriander, cumin, pepper and stir well.

5. Softly cook for about 5 minutes over medium-high heat until the vegetables are tender.
6. Serve hot and enjoy!

Nutrition: Calories 47 Fat 1 g Cholesterol 0 g Carbohydrates 8 g Sugar 6 g Fiber 2 g Protein 2 g Sodium 104 mg Calcium 36 mg Phosphorus 52 mg Potassium 298 mg

10. Appetizing Rice Salad

Preparation Time: 20 minutes

Cooking Time: 1 hour

Servings: 8

Ingredients:

- 1 cup wild rice
- 2 cups water
- 1 tablespoon olive oil
- 2/3 cup walnuts, chopped
- 1 (4 inches) celery rib, sliced
- 4 scallions, thinly sliced
- 1 medium red apple, cored and diced
- ½ cup pomegranate seeds
- ½ tablespoon lemon zest
- 3 tablespoons lemon juice
- Black pepper
- 1/3 cup olive oil

Directions:

1. In a big pot place the wild strained rice together with water and olive oil.
2. Bring to a boil and simmer for about 50 minutes until rice is tender.
3. In a mixing bowl add celery, walnuts, apple, scallions, pomegranate seeds and lemon zest.
4. Mix well with a blender the lemon juice, pepper, and olive oil.

5. Spread half of this dressing on the apple mixture and mix well.
6. When the rice is cooked, let it cool and incorporate with the fruit mixture
7. Season with the remaining dressing.
8. Serve at room temperature and enjoy!

Nutrition: Calories 300 Fat 19 g Cholesterol 0 mg Carbohydrates 34 g Sugar 11 g Fiber 5 g Protein 6 g Sodium 6 mg Calcium 30 mg Phosphorus 144 mg Potassium 296 mg

DINNER

11. Spicy Chili Crackers

Preparation Time: 15 minutes

Cooking Time: 60 minutes

Servings: 30 crackers

Ingredients:

- ¾ cup almond flour
- ¼ cup coconut four
- ¼ cup coconut flour
- ½ teaspoon paprika
- ½ teaspoon cumin
- 1 ½ teaspoons chili pepper spice
- 1 teaspoon onion powder
- ½ teaspoon sunflower seeds
- 1 whole egg
- ¼ cup unsalted almond butter

Directions:

1. Preheat your oven to 350 degrees F.
2. Line a baking sheet with parchment paper and keep it on the side.
3. Add ingredients to your food processor and pulse until you have a nice dough.
4. Divide dough into two equal parts.

5. Place one ball on a sheet of parchment paper and cover with another sheet; roll it out.
6. Cut into crackers and repeat with the other ball.
7. Transfer the prepped dough to a baking tray and bake for 8-10 minutes.
8. Remove from oven and serve.
9. Enjoy!

Nutrition: Carbs: 2.8g Fiber: 1g Protein: 1.6g Fat: 4.1g

12. Spicy Cabbage Dish

Preparation Time: 10 minutes

Cooking Time: 4 hours

Servings: 4

Ingredients:

- 2 yellow onions, chopped
- 10 cups red cabbage, shredded
- 1 cup plums, pitted and chopped
- 1 teaspoon cinnamon powder
- 1 garlic clove, minced
- 1 teaspoon cumin seeds
- ¼ teaspoon cloves, ground
- 2 tablespoons red wine vinegar
- 1 teaspoon coriander seeds
- ½ cup water

Directions:

1. Add cabbage, onion, plums, garlic, cumin, cinnamon, cloves, vinegar, coriander and water to your Slow Cooker.
2. Stir well.
3. Place lid and cook on LOW for 4 hours.
4. Divide between serving platters.
5. Enjoy!

Nutrition: Calories: 197 Fat: 1g Carbohydrates: 14g Protein: 3g Phosphorus: 115mg Potassium: 119mg Sodium: 75mg

13. Extreme Balsamic Chicken

Preparation Time: 10 minutes

Cooking Time: 35 minutes

Servings: 4

Ingredients:

- 3 boneless chicken breasts, skinless
- Sunflower seeds to taste
- ¼ cup almond flour
- 2/3 cups low-fat chicken broth
- 1 ½ teaspoons arrowroot
- ½ cup low sugar raspberry preserve
- 1 ½ tablespoons balsamic vinegar

Directions:

1. Cut chicken breast into bite-sized pieces and season them with seeds.
2. Dredge the chicken pieces in flour and shake off any excess.
3. Take a non-stick skillet and place it over medium heat.
4. Add chicken to the skillet and cook for 15 minutes, making sure to turn them half-way through.
5. Remove chicken and transfer to platter.
6. Add arrowroot, broth, raspberry preserve to the skillet and stir.

7. Stir in balsamic vinegar and reduce heat to low, stir-cook for a few minutes.

8. Transfer the chicken back to the sauce and cook for 15 minutes more.

9. Serve and enjoy!

Nutrition: Calories: 546 Fat: 35g Carbohydrates: 11g Protein: 44g Phosphorus: 120mg Potassium: 117mg Sodium: 85mg

14. Enjoyable Green lettuce and Bean Medley

Preparation Time: 10 minutes

Cooking Time: 4 hours

Servings: 4

Ingredients:

- 5 carrots, sliced
- 1 ½ cups great northern beans, dried
- 2 garlic cloves, minced
- 1 yellow onion, chopped
- Pepper to taste
- ½ teaspoon oregano, dried
- 5 ounces baby green lettuce
- 4 ½ cups low sodium veggie stock
- 2 teaspoons lemon peel, grated
- 3 tablespoon lemon juice

Directions:

1. Add beans, onion, carrots, garlic, oregano and stock to your Slow Cooker.
2. Stir well.
3. Place lid and cook on HIGH for 4 hours.
4. Add green lettuce, lemon juice and lemon peel.
5. Stir and let it sit for 5 minutes.

6. Divide between serving platters and enjoy!

Nutrition: Calories: 219 Fat: 8g Carbohydrates: 14g Protein: 8g Phosphorus: 210mg Potassium: 217mg Sodium: 85mg

MAIN DISHES

15. Quinoa & Beans Burgers

Preparation Time: 15 minutes

Cooking Time: 55 minutes

Servings: 12

Ingredients:

- ½ cup dry quinoa
- 1½ cups water
- 1 cup cooked corn kernels
- 1 (15 oz.) can black beans, drained
- 1 small boiled potato, peeled
- 1 small onion, chopped
- ½ teaspoon fresh ginger, grated finely
- 1 teaspoon garlic, minced
- ½ cup fresh cilantro, chopped
- 1 teaspoon flax meal
- 1 teaspoon ground cumin
- 1 teaspoon paprika
- 1 teaspoon chili flakes
- ½ teaspoon ground turmeric
- Salt, to taste
- Freshly ground black pepper, to taste

Directions:

1. In a pan, add water and quinoa on high heat and provide to a boil.
2. Lower the heat to medium and simmer for around 15-twenty or so minutes.
3. Drain excess water.
4. Set the oven to 375°F. Line a sizable baking sheet that has a parchment paper.
5. In a sizable bowl, add quinoa and remaining ingredients.
6. With a fork, mix till well combined.
7. Make equal-sized patties from the mixture.
8. Arrange the patties onto the prepared baking sheet in the single layer.
9. Bake for around 20-25 minutes.
10. Carefully, alter the side and cook for about 8-10 minutes.

Nutrition: Calories: 400 Fat: 9g Carbohydrates: 27g Fiber: 12gProtein: 38g

16. Veggie Balls

Preparation Time: 15 minutes

Cooking Time: 25 minutes

Servings: 5-6

Ingredients:

- 2 medium carrots, cubed into ½-inch size
- 2 tablespoons coconut almond milk
- 1 cup fresh kale leaves, trimmed and chopped
- 1 medium shallot, chopped finely
- 1 tsp. ground cumin
- ½ teaspoon granulated garlic
- ¼ tsp. ground turmeric
- Salt, to taste
- Freshly ground black pepper, to taste
- Ground flax seeds, as required

Directions:

1. Set the oven to 400°F. Line a baking sheet with parchment paper.
2. In a pan of water, arrange a steamer basket.
3. Bring the sweet potato in a steamer basket and steam approximately 10-15 minutes.
4. In a sizable bowl, put the sweet potato.
5. Add coconut almond milk and mash well.
6. Add remaining ingredients except for flax seeds and mix till well combined.
7. Make about 1½-2-inch balls from your mixture.

8. Arrange the balls onto the prepared baking sheet inside a single layer.

9. Sprinkle with flax seeds.

Bake for around 20-25 minutes.

Nutrition: Calories: 464 Fat: 12g Carbohydrates: 20g Fiber: 8g Protein: 27g

SNACKS

17. Creamy jalapeno corn

Preparation time: 5 minutes

Cooking time: 15 minutes

Servings: 2

Ingredients

- Corn kernels, fresh – 1 cup
- Red bell pepper, diced - .25 cup
- Jalapeno, seeded and diced – 1
- Cream cheese – 1.5 ounces
- Olive oil – 1 tablespoon
- Black pepper, ground - .25 teaspoon
- Cheddar cheese, low-sodium - .25 cup

Directions

1. Preheat your oven to a Fahrenheit temperature of three-hundred and fifty degrees.

2. In a medium saucepan, sauté the bell pepper and jalapeno in the olive oil until softened, about four minutes. Add in the cream cheese and continue to stir until it melts and combines with the vegetables.

3. Add in the corn, black pepper, and half of the cheese. After the mixture is combined, sprinkle the remaining

cheese over the top and place the saucepan in the oven to cook until it is hot and bubbling about fifteen minutes.

Nutrition: calories in individual servings: 284 protein grams: 7 phosphorus milligrams: 200 potassium milligrams: 293 sodium milligrams: 82 fat grams: 19 total carbohydrates grams: 20 net carbohydrates grams: 18

18. Crispy parmesan cauliflower

Preparation time: 5 minutes

Cooking time: 30 minutes

Servings: 2

Ingredients

- Cauliflower florets – 2 cups
- Black pepper, ground - .125 teaspoon
- Garlic, minced – 2 cloves
- Parmesan cheese, grated – 2 tablespoons
- Bread crumbs, plain - .25 cup
- Olive oil – 1 tablespoon

Directions

1. Preheat your oven to a Fahrenheit temperature of four-hundred degrees and line a baking sheet with kitchen parchment.

2. In one small bowl, combine the olive oil and the garlic. In another, combine the parmesan cheese, bread crumbs, and black pepper.

3. Dip the cauliflower piece-by-piece first into the olive oil mixture, and then into the bread crumb mixture. After you coat each piece, set it on the kitchen parchment-lined sheet.

4. Place the cauliflower sheet in the middle of the oven and roast the cauliflower until it reaches golden brown

perfection, about thirty minutes. Serve it immediately, while it is still warm and crispy.

Nutrition: calories in individual servings: 106 protein grams: 5 phosphorus milligrams: 166 potassium milligrams: 369 sodium milligrams: 222 fat grams: 9 total carbohydrates grams: 16 net carbohydrates grams: 14

19. Cucumber dill salad with Greek yogurt dressing

Preparation time: 5 minutes

Cooking time: 0 minute

Servings: 2

Ingredients

- Cucumbers, cut thinly – 2
- Red onion, small, thinly sliced - .5
- Greek yogurt, plain – 3 tablespoons
- Honey – 2 teaspoons
- White vinegar – 4 teaspoons
- Black pepper, ground - .125 teaspoon
- Garlic powder - .125 teaspoon
- Dill, fresh, chopped – 1.5 tablespoons

Directions

1. Use either a knife or a mandolin to cut the cucumbers into thin and even slices, about .25 of an inch thick.

2. In a medium bowl, whisk together the fresh dill, garlic powder, black pepper, white vinegar, honey, and greek yogurt.

3. Into the bowl with the prepared greek yogurt dressing, add the cucumbers and red onion, and toss them together until fully coated. Cover the bowl with a lid or plastic wrap and allow it to chill in the fridge for at

least an hour before enjoying. You can make this salad up to a day in advance.

Nutrition: calories in individual servings: 106 protein grams: 5 phosphorus milligrams: 166 potassium milligrams: 369 sodium milligrams: 222 fat grams: 9 total carbohydrates grams: 16 net carbohydrates grams: 14

20. Zesty green beans with almonds

Preparation time: 5 minutes

Cooking time: 10 minutes

Servings: 2

Ingredients

- Green beans, trimmed - .5 pound
- Olive oil – 1 tablespoon
- Shallot, diced – 1
- Garlic, minced – 2 cloves
- Almonds, sliced – 2 tablespoons
- Lemon zest - .25 teaspoon
- Lemon juice – 1 teaspoon
- Black pepper, ground - .125 teaspoon

Directions

1. In a large skillet, sauté the shallot and garlic in the olive oil over medium heat until soft, about three minutes. Add in the green beans and black pepper and continue to cook the green beans until they are tender about seven minutes.

2. Once the green beans are ready, stir in the lemon juice and lemon zest, and then top the skillet off with the sliced almonds.

Nutrition: calories in individual servings: 143 protein grams: 3 phosphorus milligrams: 84 potassium milligrams: 322 sodium milligrams: 8 fat grams: 10 total carbohydrates grams: 11 net carbohydrates grams: 8

SOUP AND STEW

21. Pesto Green Vegetable Soup

Preparation Time: 10 minutes

Cooking Time: 15 minutes

Servings: 1

Ingredients:

- 2 teaspoons olive oil
- 1 sliced leek, white and light green
- 2 celery stalks, diced
- 1 teaspoon minced garlic
- 2 cups sodium-free chicken stock
- 1 cup chopped snow peas
- 1 tablespoon chopped fresh thyme
- Juice and zest of ½ lemon
- ¼ teaspoon freshly ground black pepper
- 1 tablespoon Basil Pesto

Directions:

1. Add olive oil in a large saucepan.
2. Add the leek, celery, and garlic, and sauté until tender, about 3 minutes.
3. Stir in the stock and bring to a boil.

4. Stir in the snow peas, and thyme, and simmer for about 5 minutes.

5. Remove the pan from the heat, and stir in the lemon juice, lemon zest, pepper, and pesto.

6. Serve immediately.

Nutrition: Calories: 170 Fat: 13g Carbohydrates: 8g Protein: 3g Sodium: 333mg Phosphorus: 42mg Potassium: 200mg

22. Easy Low-Sodium Chicken Broth

Preparation Time: 10 minutes

Cooking Time: 4 hours

Servings: 1

Ingredients:

- 2 pounds skinless whole chicken, cut into pieces
- 4 garlic cloves, lightly crushed
- 2 celery stalks, with greens, roughly chopped
- 2 carrots, roughly chopped
- 1 sweet onion, cut into quarters
- 10 peppercorns
- 4 fresh thyme sprigs
- 2 bay leaves
- Water

Directions:

1. In a large stockpot, place the chicken, garlic, celery, carrots, onion, peppercorns, thyme, and bay leaves, and cover with water by about 3 inches.
2. Let the water boil over high heat. Simmer for about 4 hours in low heat.
3. Skim off any foam on top of the stock and pour the stock through a fine-mesh sieve.
4. Pick off all the usable chicken meat for another recipe, discard the bones and other solids, and allow the stock

to cool for about 30 minutes before transferring it to sealable containers.

5. You can put the stock in the refrigerator for 1 week or up to 2 months in the freezer.

Nutrition: Calories: 32 Carbohydrates: 8g Protein: 1g Sodium: 57mg Potassium: 187mg Phosphorus: 50mg

23. Cream of pepper Soup

Preparation Time: 15 minutes

Cooking Time: 30 minutes

Servings: 4

Ingredients:

- 1 tablespoon olive oil
- ½ sweet onion, chopped
- 2 teaspoons minced garlic
- 4 cups fresh pepper
- ¼ cup chopped fresh parsley
- 3 cups of water
- ¼ cup heavy (whipping) cream
- 1 tablespoon freshly squeezed lemon juice
- Freshly ground black pepper

Directions:

1. On a heated olive oil, sauté the onion and garlic in a large saucepan for 3 minutes.

2. Add the pepper and parsley, and sauté for 5 minutes.

3. Stir in the water, bring to a boil, then reduce the heat to low. Simmer the soup until the vegetables are tender, about 20 minutes.

4. Let it cool for 5 minutes, then, along with the heavy cream, purée the soup in batches in a food processor (or a blender or a handheld immersion blender).

5. Return the soup to the pot and cook through on low heat.

6. Add the lemon juice, season with pepper, and stir to combine. Serve hot.

Nutrition: Calories: 141 Fat: 14g Carbohydrates: 3g Protein: 2g

Sodium: 36mg Phosphorus: 38mg Potassium: 200mg

24. Vegetable Minestrone

Preparation Time: 20 minutes

Cooking Time: 20 minutes

Servings: 6

Ingredients:

- 1 teaspoon olive oil
- ½ sweet onion, chopped
- 1 celery stalk, diced
- 1 teaspoon minced garlic
- 2 cups sodium-free chicken stock
- 1 zucchini, diced
- ½ cup shredded stemmed kale
- Freshly ground black pepper
- 1-ounce grated Parmesan cheese

Directions:

1. Prepare a large saucepan over medium-high heat.
2. Add the onion, celery, and garlic. Sauté until softened, about 5 minutes.
3. Stir in the stock, zucchini, and bring to a boil. Let it simmer for 15 minutes.
4. Stir in the kale and season with pepper.
5. Garnish with the parmesan cheese and serve.

Nutrition: Calories: 100 Fat: 3g Carbohydrates: 6g Protein: 4g Sodium: 195mg Phosphorus: 70mg Potassium: 200mg

25. Vibrant Carrot Soup

Preparation Time: 15 minutes

Cooking Time: 25 minutes

Servings: 4

Ingredients:

- 1 tablespoon olive oil
- ½ sweet onion, chopped
- 2 teaspoons grated peeled fresh ginger
- 1 teaspoon minced fresh garlic
- 4 cups of water
- 3 carrots, chopped
- 1 teaspoon ground turmeric
- ½ cup of coconut milk
- 1 tablespoon chopped fresh cilantro

Directions:

1. Heat the olive oil in a saucepan.
2. Sauté the onion, ginger, and garlic until softened.
3. Stir in the water, carrots, and turmeric. Bring the soup to a boil, reduce the heat to low, and simmer until the carrots are tender about 20 minutes.
4. Transfer the soup in batches to a food processor (or blender) and process with the coconut milk until the soup is smooth.

5. Reheat the soup in a pan.

6. Serve topped with the cilantro.

Nutrition: Calories: 113 Fat: 10g Protein: 1g Carbohydrates: 7g Sodium: 30mg Phosphorus: 50mg Potassium: 200mg;

VEGETABLE

26. Lime Green lettuce and Chickpeas Salad

Preparation Time: 10 minutes

Cooking Time: 0 minutes

Servings: 4

Ingredients:

- 16 ounces canned chickpeas, drained and rinsed
- 2 cups baby green lettuce leaves
- ½ tablespoon lime juice
- 2 tablespoons olive oil
- 1 teaspoon cumin, ground
- Sea salt and black pepper
- ½ teaspoon chili flakes

Directions:

1. In a bowl, mix the chickpeas with the green lettuce and the rest of the ingredients, toss and serve cold.

Nutrition: Calories 240, Fat 8.2, Fiber 5.3, Carbs 11.6, Protein 12

27. Fried Rice with Kale

Preparation Time: 10 minutes

Cooking Time: 12 minutes

Servings: 4

Ingredients:

- 2 tbsp. Extra virgin oil
- 8 oz. Tofu, chopped
- 6 Scallion, white and green parts, thinly sliced
- 2 cups Kale, stemmed and chopped
- 3 cups Cooked white rice
- ¼ cup Stir fry sauce

Directions:

1. In a huge skillet on medium-high heat, warm the oil until it shimmers.
2. Add the tofu, scallions, and kale. Cook for 5 to 7 minutes, frequently stirring, until the vegetables are soft.
3. Add the white rice and stir-fry sauce. Cook for 3 to 5 minutes, occasionally stirring, until heated through.

Nutrition: Calories: 301 Total Fat: 11g Total Carbs: 36g Sugar: 1g Fiber: 3g Protein: 16g Sodium: 2,535mg

28. Stir-Fried Gingery Veggies

Preparation Time: 10 minutes

Cooking Time: 10 minutes

Servings: 4

Ingredients:

- 1 tablespoon oil
- 3 cloves of garlic, minced
- 1 onion, chopped
- 1 thumb-size ginger, sliced
- 1 tablespoon water
- 1 large carrots, peeled and julienned and seedless
- 1 large green bell pepper, julienned and seedless
- 1 large yellow bell pepper, julienned and seedless
- 1 large red bell pepper, julienned and seedless
- 1 zucchini, julienned
- Salt and pepper to taste

Directions:

1. Heat oil in a nonstick saucepan over a high flame and sauté the garlic, onion, and ginger until fragrant.
2. Stir in the rest of the ingredients.
3. Keep on stirring for at least 5 minutes until vegetables are tender.
4. Serve and enjoy.

Nutrition: Calories 70 Total Fat 4g Saturated Fat 1g Total Carbs 9g Net Carbs 7g Protein 1g Sugar: 4g Fiber 2g Sodium 173mg Potassium 163mg

29. Minty Olives Salad

Preparation time: 10 minutes

Cooking time: 0 minutes

Servings: 4

Ingredients:

- 1 cup kalamata olives, pitted and sliced
- 1 cup black olives, pitted and halved
- 1 red onion, chopped
- 2 tablespoons oregano, chopped
- 1 tablespoon mint, chopped
- 2 tablespoons balsamic vinegar
- ¼ cup olive oil
- 2 teaspoons Italian herbs, dried
- A pinch of sea salt and black pepper

Directions:

1. In a salad bowl, mix the olives and the rest of the ingredients, toss and serve cold.

Nutrition: calories 190, fat 8.1, fiber 5.8, carbs 11.6, protein 4.6 Phosphorus: 110mg Potassium: 117mg Sodium: 75mg

SIDE DISHES

30. Salmon chowder

Preparation time: 20 minutes

Cooking time: 4 hours

Servings: 2

Ingredients

- 3 pounds salmon fillets, sliced into manageable pieces
- 1 1/2 cups onion, chopped
- 2 potatoes, cubed – limit this
- 3 cups water
- 1/3 teaspoon pepper
- 18-ounce evaporated milk, non-fat

Directions

1. Put together onion, salmon, potatoes, and pepper in the slow cooker. Pour water
2. Cover and cook for 8 hours on low. Secure the lid.
3. After the 8-hour cooking cycle, turn off the heat. Adjust seasoning according to your preferred taste.
4. Stir in milk. Cover and cook for another 30 minutes. Serve right away.

Nutrition: protein: 33.8 g potassium: 204.3 mg sodium: 183.5 mg

SALAD

31. Cucumber Couscous Salad

Preparation Time: 5 minutes

Cooking Time: 0 minutes

Servings: 4

Ingredients:

- 1 cucumber, sliced
- ½ cup red bell pepper, sliced
- ¼ cup sweet onion, sliced
- ¼ cup parsley, chopped
- ½ cup couscous, cooked
- 2 tablespoons olive oil
- 2 tablespoons rice vinegar
- 2 tablespoons feta cheese crumbled
- 1 ½ teaspoon dried basil
- 1/4 teaspoon black pepper

Direction:

1. Put all the salad ingredients into a suitable salad bowl.
2. Toss them well and refrigerate for 1 hour.
3. Serve.

Nutrition: Calories 202 Total Fat 9.8g Sodium 258mg Protein 6.2g Calcium 80mg Phosphorous 192mg Potassium 209mg

32. Carrot Jicama Salad

Preparation Time: 5 minutes

Cooking Time: 0 minutes

Servings: 2

Ingredients:

- 2 cup carrots, julienned
- 1 1/2 cups jicama, julienned
- 2 tablespoons lime juice
- 1 tablespoon olive oil
- ½ tablespoon apple cider
- ½ teaspoon brown Swerve

Direction:

1. Put all the salad ingredients into a suitable salad bowl.
2. Toss them well and refrigerate for 1 hour.
3. Serve.

Nutrition: Calories 173 Total Fat 7.1g Sodium 80mg Protein 1.6g Calcium 50mg Phosphorous 96mg Potassium 501mg

FISH & SEAFOOD

33. Thai tuna wraps

Preparation time: 10 minutes

Cooking time: 0 minute

Servings: 4

Ingredients

- ¼ cup unsalted peanut butter
- 2 tablespoons freshly squeezed lemon juice
- 1 teaspoon low-sodium soy sauce
- ½ teaspoon ground ginger
- 1/8 teaspoon cayenne pepper
- 1 (6-ounce) can no-salt-added or low-sodium chunk light tuna, drained
- 1 cup shredded red cabbage
- 2 scallions, white and green parts, chopped
- 1 cup grated carrots
- 8 butter lettuce leaves

Directions

1. In a medium bowl, stir together the peanut butter, lemon juice, soy sauce, ginger, and cayenne pepper until well combined.

2. Stir in the tuna, cabbage, scallions, and carrots.

3. Divide the tuna filling evenly between the butter lettuce leaves and serve.

Nutrition: per serving: calories: 175; total fat; 10g; saturated fat: 1g; sodium: 98mg; potassium: 421mg; phosphorus: 153mg; carbohydrates: 8g; fiber: 2g; protein: 17g; sugar: 4g

34. Grilled fish and vegetable packets

Preparation time: 15 minutes

Cooking time: 12 minutes

Servings: 4

Ingredients

- 1 (8-ounce) package sliced mushrooms
- 1 leek, white and green parts, chopped
- 1 cup frozen corn
- 4 (4-ounce) atlantic cod fillets
- Juice of 1 lemon
- 3 tablespoons olive oil

Directions

1. Prepare and preheat the grill to medium coals and set a grill 6 inches from the coals.

2. Tear off four 30-inch long strips of heavy-duty aluminum foil.

3. Arrange the mushrooms, leek, and corn in the center of each piece of foil and top with the fish.

4. Drizzle the packet contents evenly with the lemon juice and olive oil.

5. Bring the longer length sides of the foil together at the top and, holding the edges together, fold them over twice and then fold in the width sides to form a sealed packet with room for the steam.

6. Put the packets on the grill and grill for 10 to 12 minutes until the vegetables are tender-crisp and the fish flakes when tested with a fork. Be careful opening the packets because the escaping steam can be scalding.

Nutrition: per serving: calories: 267; total fat: 12g; saturated fat: 2g; sodium: 97mg; potassium: 582mg; phosphorus: 238mg; carbohydrates: 13g; fiber: 2g; protein: 29g; sugar: 3g

35. Lemon butter salmon

Preparation time: 15 minutes

Cooking time: 15 minutes

Servings: 6

Ingredients

- 1 tablespoon butter
- 2 tablespoons olive oil
- 1 tablespoon dijon mustard
- 1 tablespoons lemon juice
- 2 cloves garlic, crushed
- 1 teaspoon dried dill
- 1 teaspoon dried basil leaves
- 1 tablespoon capers
- 24-ounce salmon filet

Directions

1. Put all of the ingredients except the salmon in a saucepan over medium heat.
2. Bring to a boil and then simmer for 5 minutes.
3. Preheat your grill.
4. Create a packet using foil.
5. Place the sauce and salmon inside.
6. Seal the packet.
7. Grill for 12 minutes.

Nutrition: calories 292 protein 22 g carbohydrates 2 g fat 22 g cholesterol 68 mg sodium 190 mg potassium 439 mg phosphorus 280 mg calcium 21 mg

36. Crab cake

Preparation time: 15 minutes

Cooking time: 9 minutes

Servings: 6

Ingredients

- 1/4 cup onion, chopped
- 1/4 cup bell pepper, chopped
- 1 egg, beaten
- 6 low-sodium crackers, crushed
- 1/4 cup low-fat mayonnaise
- 1-pound crab meat
- 1 tablespoon dry mustard
- Pepper to taste
- 2 tablespoons lemon juice
- 1 tablespoon fresh parsley
- 1 tablespoon garlic powder
- 3 tablespoons olive oil

Directions

1. Mix all the ingredients except the oil.
2. Form 6 patties from the mixture.
3. Pour the oil into a pan in a medium heat.
4. Cook the crab cakes for 5 minutes.
5. Flip and cook for another 4 minutes.

Nutrition: calories 189 protein 13 g carbohydrates 5 g fat 14 g cholesterol 111 mg sodium 342 mg potassium 317 mg phosphorus 185 mg calcium 52 mg fiber 0.5 g

37. Baked fish in cream sauce

Preparation time: 10 minutes

Cooking time: 40 minutes

Servings: 4

Ingredients

- 1-pound haddock
- 1/2 cup all-purpose flour
- 2 tablespoons butter (unsalted)
- 1/4 teaspoon pepper
- 2 cups fat-free nondairy creamer
- 1/4 cup water

Directions

1. Preheat your oven to 350 degrees f.
2. Spray baking pan with oil.
3. Sprinkle with a little flour.
4. Arrange fish on the pan
5. Season with pepper.
6. Sprinkle remaining flour on the fish.
7. Spread creamer on both sides of the fish.
8. Bake for 40 minutes or until golden.
9. Spread cream sauce on top of the fish before serving.

Nutrition: calories 383 protein 24 g carbohydrates 46 g fat 11 g cholesterol 79 mg sodium 253 mg potassium 400 mg phosphorus 266 mg calcium 46 mg fiber 0.4 g

38. Turkey & Pumpkin Chili

Preparation Time: 15 minutes

Cooking Time: 41 minutes

Servings: 4-6

Ingredients:

- 2 tablespoons extra-virgin olive oil
- 1 green bell pepper, seeded and chopped
- 1 small yellow onion, chopped
- 2 garlic cloves, chopped finely
- 1-pound lean ground turkey
- 1 (15-ounce) pumpkin puree
- 1 (14 ½-ounce) can diced Red bell peppers with liquid
- 1 teaspoon ground cumin
- ½ teaspoon ground turmeric
- ½ teaspoon ground cinnamon
- 1 cup of water
- 1 can chickpeas, rinsed and drained

Directions:

1. Heat-up oil on medium-low heat in a big pan. Add the bell pepper, onion, and garlic and sauté for approximately 5 minutes. Add turkey and cook for about 5-6 minutes.
2. Add Red bell peppers, pumpkin, spices, and water and convey to your boil on high heat. Reduce the

temperature to medium-low heat and stir in chickpeas. Simmer, covered for approximately a half-hour, stirring occasionally. Serve hot.

Nutrition: Calories: 437 Fat: 17g Carbohydrates: 29g Protein: 42g Phosphorus 150 mg Potassium 652 mg Sodium 570 mg

39. Chicken curry

Preparation Time: 10 minutes

Cooking Time: 4 minutes

Servings: 4

Ingredients

- 1lb skinless chicken breasts
- 1 medium onion, thinly sliced
- 1 15 ounce can chickpeas, drained and rinsed well
- ½ cup light coconut almond milk
- ½ cup chicken stock (see recipe)
- 1 15ounce can sodium-free tomato sauce
- 2 tablespoon curry powder
- 1 teaspoon low-sodium salt
- ½ cayenne powder
- 1 cup green peas
- 2 tablespoon lemon juice

Directions

1. Place the chicken breasts, onion, chickpeas into a 4 to 6-quart slow cooker.

2. Mix the coconut almond milk, chicken stock, tomato sauce, curry powder, salt, and cayenne together and pour into the slow cooker, stirring to coat well.

3. Cover and cook on low for 8 hours or high for 4 hours.

4. Stir in the peas and lemon juice 5 minutes before serving.

Nutrition: calories 302, fat 5g, carbs 43g, protein 24g, fiber 9g, potassium 573mg, sodium 800mg

40. Lemon & herb turkey breasts

Preparation Time: 25 minutes

Cooking Time: 3 1/2 hours

Servings: 12

Ingredients

- 1 can (14-1/2 ounces) chicken broth
- 1/2 cup lemon juice
- 1/4 cup packed brown sugar
- 1/4 cup fresh sage
- 1/4 cup fresh thyme leaves
- 1/4 cup lime juice
- 1/4 cup cider vinegar
- 1/4 cup olive oil
- 1 envelope low-sodium onion soup mix
- 2 tablespoon dijon mustard
- 1 tablespoon fresh marjoram, minced
- 1 teaspoon paprika
- 1 teaspoon garlic powder
- 1 teaspoon pepper
- ½ teaspoon low-sodium salt
- 2 2lb boneless skinless turkey breast halves

Directions

1. Make a marinade by blending all the ingredients in a blender.

2. Pour over the turkey and leave overnight.

3. Place the turkey and marinade in a 4 to 6-quart slow cooker and cover.

4. Cover and cook on high for 3-1/2 to 4-1/2 hours or until a thermometer reads 165°.

Nutrition: calories 219, fat 5g, carbs 3g, protein 36g, fiber 0g, potassium 576mg, sodium 484mg

41. Beef chimichangas

Preparation Time: 10minutes

Cooking Time: 10-12 hours

Servings: 16

Ingredients

- Shredded beef
- 3lb boneless beef chuck roast, fat trimmed away
- 3 tablespoon low-sodium taco seasoning mix
- 1 10ounce canned low-sodium diced Red bell peppers
- 6ounce canned diced green chilies with the juice
- 3 garlic cloves, minced
- To serve
- 16 medium flour tortillas
- Sodium-free refried beans
- Mexican rice, sour cream, cheddar cheese
- Guacamole, salsa, lettuce

Directions

1. Arrange the beef in a 5-quart or larger slow cooker.
2. Sprinkle over taco seasoning and coat well.
3. Add Red bell peppers and garlic and cover.
4. Cook on low for 10 to 12 hours.
5. When cooked remove the beef and shred.

6. Make burritos out of the shredded beef, refried beans, Mexican rice, and cheese.

7. Bake for 10 minutes at 350° f until brown.

8. Serve with salsa, lettuce, and guacamole.

Nutrition: calories 249, fat 18g, carbs 3g, protein 33g, fiber 5g, potassium 633mg, sodium 457mg

MEAT RECIPES

42. Beef Pot Roast

Preparation Time: 20 minutes

Cooking Time: 1 hour

Servings: 3

Ingredients

- Round bone roast

- 2 - 4 pounds chuck roast

Directions:

1. Trim off excess fat

2. Place a tablespoon of oil in a large skillet and heat to medium

3. Roll pot roast in flour and brown on all sides in a hot skillet

4. After the meat gets a brown color, reduce heat to low

5. Season with pepper and herbs and add 1/2 cup of water

6. Cook slowly for 11/2 hours or until it looks ready

Nutrition: Calories 157 Protein 24 g Fat 13 g Carbs 0 g Phosphorus 204 mg Sodium (Na) 50 mg

43. Slow-cooked Beef Brisket

Preparation Time: 10 minutes

Cooking Time: 3 hours and 30 minutes

Servings: 6

Ingredients

- 10-ounce chuck roast
- 1 onion, sliced
- 1 cup carrots, peeled and sliced
- 1 tablespoon mustard
- 1 tablespoon thyme (fresh or dried)
- 1 tablespoon rosemary (fresh or dried)
- 2 garlic cloves
- 2 tablespoon extra-virgin olive oil
- 1 teaspoon black pepper
- 1 cup homemade chicken stock (p.52)
- 1 cup water

Directions

1. Preheat oven to 300°f/150°c/Gas Mark 2.
2. Trim any fat from the beef and soak vegetables in warm water.
3. Make a paste by mixing together the mustard, thyme, rosemary, and garlic, before mixing in the oil and pepper.

4. Combine this mix with the stock.

5. Pour the mixture over the beef into an oven proof baking dish.

6. Place the vegetables onto the bottom of the baking dish with the beef.

7. Cover and roast for 3 hours, or until tender.

8. Uncover the dish and continue to cook for 30 minutes in the oven.

9. Serve hot!

Nutrition: Calories: 151 Fat: 7g Carbohydrates: 7g Phosphorus: 144mg Potassium: 344mg Sodium: 279mg Protein: 15g

BROTHS, CONDIMENT AND SEASONING

44. Classic Spice Blend

Preparation Time: 10 minutes

Cooking Time: 0 minutes

Servings: 2 tbsp.

Ingredients:

- 1 tablespoon whole black peppercorns
- 2 teaspoons caraway seeds
- 2 teaspoons celery seeds
- 1 teaspoon dill seeds
- 1 teaspoon cumin seeds

Directions:

1. Grind the peppercorns, caraway seeds, celery seeds, dill seeds, and cumin in a spice blender or a mortar and pestle. Grind until the seeds are broken down, and the mixture almost becomes a powder.

Nutrition: Calories: 2 Fat: 0g Sodium: 0mg Phosphorus: 3mg Potassium: 8mg Carbohydrates: 0g Protein: 0g

45. Basil Pesto Sauce

Preparation Time: 15 minutes

Cooking Time: 0 minutes

Servings: 1

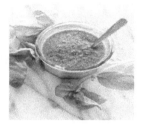

Ingredients:

- 2/3 cup of nutritional yeast
- .5 of a fresh lemon
- 6 tsp oil (olive)
- 3 garlic cloves
- 1 tsp of pepper
- 6 tsp of flax oil
- 16 oz. basil leaves
- 8 oz. of pine nuts

Directions:

1. Extract juice out of lemon and put all of the items into a food processor except olive and flax oil.
2. Mix the oils and pour them into the processor through the top to evenly distribute them while blending all of the ingredients.

3. Stir from the bottom of the blender as needed. Store prepared pesto sauce in a jar or covered container until ready to use.

Nutrition: Calories 122 Phosphorus 99 mg Protein 4 g Carbohydrates 4 g Sodium 7 g Potassium 158 mg Fat 10 g

46. Seafood Seasoning

Preparation Time: 15 minutes

Cooking Time: 0 minutes

Servings: 1

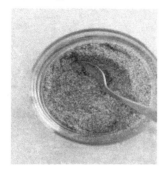

Ingredients:

- 5 tsp of fennel seeds
- 4 tsp of dried parsley
- 5 tsp of dried basil
- 1 tsp of dried lemon peel

Directions:

1. Crush up the fennel seeds and put the rest of the items into a jar, shaking to mix. Keep sealed until ready to coat fish or seafood.

Nutrition: Calories 10 Phosphorus 13 mg Protein 0 g Carbohydrates 2 g Sodium 4 mg Potassium 65 mg Fat 0 g

DRINKS AND SMOOTHIES

47. Citrus Smoothie

Preparation Time: 5 minutes

Cooking Time: 2 minutes

Servings: 2

Ingredients:

- 1 large orange, peeled, halved
- ¼ lemon, peeled, seeded
- ½ cup (85 g) pineapple, peeled, cubed
- ¼ cup (60 g) frozen mango
- 1 cup (130 g) ice cubes

Directions:

1. Prepare all ingredients into the container and secure lid.
2. Turn machine on and slowly increase speed to high.
3. Blend for 1 minute or until the desired consistency is reached.

Nutrition: Calories: 280 Fat: 0g Carbs: 67g Protein: 4g Sodium: 30mg Potassium: 570mg Phosphorus: 0mg

48. Pineapple Protein Smoothie

Preparation Time: 5 minutes

Cooking Time:

Servings: 1

Ingredients:

- 1/2 cup cottage cheese
- 1/2 cup frozen pineapple chunks
- 1/2 tsp brown sugar (optional)
- 1/4 tsp vanilla extract
- 1 Tbsp ground flaxseed (optional)
- 1 cup milk of choice (unsweetened almond milk)

Directions:

1. Place all of the ingredients into a blender, and then blend until smooth.

2. Serve immediately.

Nutrition: Calories: 220 Carbohydrates: 29g Protein: 24g Fat: 0.5g Sodium: 195mg Potassium: 325mg Phosphorus: 0mg

DESSERT

49. Chocolate Cookies

Preparation Time: 10 minutes

Cooking Time: 10 minutes

Servings: 18

Ingredients:

- 2 eggs, lightly beaten
- 3 tbsp butter
- 3 tbsp unsweetened cocoa powder
- 1 1/2 cups almond flour
- 1 tsp vanilla
- 1/4 cup Swerve
- 3 oz unsweetened chocolate, chopped
- Pinch of salt

Directions:

1. Add chocolate, butter, and cocoa powder into the pan and melt over medium-low heat.
2. Remove from heat and set aside.
3. Add eggs, vanilla, salt, and swerve in a bowl and blend until well combined.
4. Add melted chocolate mixture into the egg mixture and mix well.

5. Add almond flour and mix until well combined. Place in refrigerator for 1 hour.

6. Preheat the oven to 325 F. Line baking tray with parchment paper and spray with cooking spray.

7. Scoop out batter onto a baking tray and bake for 10 minutes.

8. Serve and enjoy.

Nutrition: Calories 66 Fat 5 g Carbohydrates 4.9 g Sugar 3 g Protein 2 g Cholesterol 25 mg Phosphorus: 80mg Potassium: 97mg Sodium: 95mg

50. Chocolate Muffins

Preparation Time: 10 minutes

Cooking Time: 30 minutes

Servings: 10

Ingredients:

- 2 eggs, lightly beaten
- 1/2 cup cream
- 1/2 tsp vanilla
- 1 cup almond flour
- 1 tbsp baking powder, gluten-free
- 4 tbsp Swerve
- 1/2 cup unsweetened cocoa powder
- Pinch of salt

Directions:

1. Preheat the oven to 375 F.
2. Spray a muffin tray with cooking spray and set aside.
3. In a mixing bowl, mix together almond flour, baking powder, swerve, cocoa powder, and salt.
4. In a separate bowl, beat eggs with cream, and vanilla.
5. Pour egg mixture into the almond flour mixture and mix well.
6. Pour batter into the prepared muffin tray and bake in preheated oven for 30 minutes.

7. Serve and enjoy.

Nutrition: Calories 101 Fat 7.5 g Carbohydrates 6.7 g Sugar 0.4 g Protein 4.5 g Cholesterol 35 mg Phosphorus: 75mg Potassium: 57mg Sodium: 78mg

51. Roasted Up Brussels

Preapration Time:10 Minutes

Cooking Time: 15 Minutes

Servings: 4

Ingredients:

- One block Brussels sprouts
- ½ teaspoon garlic
- Two teaspoons olive oil
- ½ teaspoon pepper
- Salt as needed

Directions:

1. Pre-heat your Fryer to 390-degree F.
2. Remove leaves off the chokes, leaving only the head.
3. Wash and dry the sprouts well.
4. Make a mixture of olive oil, salt, and pepper with garlic.
5. Cover sprouts with the marinade and let them rest for 5 minutes.
6. Transfer coated sprouts to Air Fryer and cook for 15 minutes.
7. Serve and enjoy!

Nutrition: Calories: 43 Fat: 2g Carbohydrates: 5g Protein: 2g

52. Roasted Brussels and Pine Nuts

Preapration Time:10 Minutes

Cooking Time: 35 Minutes

Servings: 6

Ingredients:

- 15 ounces Brussels sprouts
- One tablespoon olive oil
- One and ¾ ounces raisins, drained
- Juice of 1 orange
- One and ¾ ounces toasted pine nuts

Directions:

1. Take a pot of boiling water, then add sprouts and boil them for 4 minutes.
2. Transfer the sprouts to cold water and drain them well.
3. Place them in a freezer and cool them.
4. Take your raisins and soak them in orange juice for 20 minutes.
5. Warm your Air Fryer to a temperature of 392-degree F.
6. Take a pan and pour oil, and stir the sprouts.
7. Take the sprouts and transfer them to your Air Fryer.
8. Roast for 15 minutes.
9. Serve the sprouts with pine nuts, orange juice, and raisins!

Nutrition: Calories: 260 Fat: 20g Carbohydrates: 10g Protein: 7g

53. Low-Calorie Beets Dish

Preapration Time:10 Minutes

Cooking Time: 10 Minutes

Servings: 2

Ingredients:

- Four whole beets
- One tablespoon balsamic vinegar
- One tablespoon olive oil
- Salt and pepper to taste
- Two springs rosemary

Directions:

1. Wash your beets and peel them
2. Cut beets into cubes
3. Take a bowl and mix in rosemary, pepper, salt, vinegar
4. Cover beets with the Directions:ared sauce
5. Coat the beets with olive oil
6. Pre-heat your Fryer to 400-degree F
7. Transfer beets to Air Fryer cooking basket and cook for 10 minutes
8. Serve with your cheese sauce and enjoy!

Nutrition: Calories: 149 Fat: 1g Carbohydrates: 5g Protein: 30g

54. Broccoli and Parmesan Dish

Preapration Time:5 Minutes

Cooking Time: 20 Minutes

Servings: 4

Ingredients:

- One fresh head broccoli
- One tablespoon olive oil
- One lemon, juiced
- Salt and pepper to taste
- 1-ounce parmesan cheese, grated

Directions:

1. Wash broccoli thoroughly and cut them into florets.
2. Add the listed Ingredients:to your broccoli and mix well.
3. Preheat your fryer to 365-degree F.
4. Air fry broccoli for 20 minutes.
5. Serve and enjoy!

Nutrition: Calories: 114 Fat: 6g Carbohydrates: 10 g Protein: 7g

55. Bacon and Asparagus Spears

Preapration Time:15 Minutes

Cooking Time: 8 Minutes

Servings: 4

Ingredients:

- 20 spears asparagus
- Four bacon slices
- One tablespoon olive oil
- One tablespoon sesame oil
- One garlic clove, crushed

Directions:

1. Warm your Air Fryer to 380 degrees F
2. Take a small bowl and add oil, crushed garlic, and mix
3. Separate asparagus into four bunches and wrap them in bacon
4. Brush wraps with oil and garlic mix, transfer to your Air Fryer basket
5. Cook for 8 minutes
6. Serve and enjoy!

Nutrition: Calories: 175 Fat: 15g Carbohydrates: 6g Protein: 5g

56. Healthy Low Carb Fish Nugget

Preapration Time:5 Minutes

Cooking Time: 10 Minutes

Servings: 4

Ingredients:

- 1-pound fresh cod
- Two tablespoons olive oil
- ½ cup almond flour
- Two larges finely beaten eggs
- 1-2 cups almond meal

Directions:

1. Preheat your Air Fryer to 388 degrees F
2. Take a food processor and add olive oil, almond meal, salt, and blend
3. Take three bowls and add almond flour, almond meal, beaten eggs individually
4. Take cods and cut them into slices of 1-inch thickness and 2-inch length
5. Dredge slices into flour, eggs, and crumbs
6. Transfer nuggets to Air Fryer cooking basket and cook for 10 minutes until golden
7. Serve and enjoy!

Nutrition: Calories: 196 Fat: 14g Carbohydrates: 6g Protein: 14g

57. Fried Up Pumpkin Seeds

Preapration Time:10 Minutes

Cooking Time: 60 Minutes

Servings: 2

Ingredients:

- One and ½ cups pumpkin seeds
- Olive oil as needed
- One and ½ teaspoons salt
- One teaspoon smoked paprika

Directions:

1. Cut pumpkin and scrape out seeds and flesh
2. Separate flesh from seeds and rinse the seeds under cold water
3. Bring two-quarter of salted water to boil and add seeds, boil for 10 minutes
4. Drain seeds and spread them on a kitchen towel
5. Dry for 20 minutes
6. Preheat your fryer to 350 degrees F
7. Take a bowl and add seeds, smoked paprika, and olive oil
8. Season with salt and transfer to your Air Fryer cooking basket
9. Cook for 35 minutes, enjoy it!

Nutrition: Calories: 237 Fat: 21g Carbohydrates: 4g Protein: 12g

58. Decisive Tiger Shrimp Platter

Preapration Time:5 Minutes

Cooking Time: 10 Minutes

Servings: 6

Ingredients:

- One ¼ pound tiger shrimp, or a count of about 16 to 20
- ¼ teaspoons cayenne pepper
- ½ teaspoons old bay seasoning
- ¼ teaspoons smoked paprika
- One tablespoon olive oil

Directions:

1. Pre-heat your Fryer to 390-degree Fahrenheit
2. Take a bowl and add the listed Ingredients:
3. Mix well
4. Transfer the shrimp to your fryer cooking basket and cook for 5 minutes
5. Remove and serve the shrimp over cauliflower rice if preferred
6. Enjoy!

Nutrition: Calories: 251 Carbohydrate: 3g Protein: 17g Fat: 19g

59. Air Fried Olives

Preapration Time:5 Minutes

Cooking Time: 8 Minutes

Servings: 4

Ingredients:

- 1 (5½-ounce / 156-g) jar pitted green olives
- ½ cup all-purpose flour
- Salt and pepper, to taste
- ½ cup bread crumbs
- One egg

Directions:

1. Preheat the air fryer oven to 400ºF (204ºC).
2. Take away the olives from the jar and dry thoroughly with paper towels.
3. In a small bowl, combine the flour with salt and pepper to taste. Place the bread crumbs in another small container. In a third small bowl, beat the egg.
4. Spray the basket with cooking spray.
5. Drench the olives in the flour, then the egg, and then the bread crumbs.
6. Place the breaded olives in the air fryer basket. It is okay to stack them. Spray the olives with cooking spray.
7. Place the air fryer basket onto the warming pan.
8. Slide into Rack Position 2.
9. Select Air Fry and set the Time to 6 minutes.

10. Flip the olives and air fry for an additional 2 minutes, or until brown and crisp.
11. Cool for 5 minutes before serving.

Nutrition: Calories: 188 Fat: 6.8g Carbs: 1.9g Protein: 30.3g

60. Bacon-Wrapped Dates

Preapration Time:10 Minutes

Cooking Time: 6 Minutes

Servings: 6

Ingredients:

- 12 dates, pitted
- Six slices of high-quality bacon, cut in half
- Cooking spray

Directions:

1. Preheat the air fryer oven to 360ºF (182ºC).
2. Covering each date with half a bacon slice and secure with a toothpick.
3. Spray the air fryer basket by means of cooking spray, then place bacon-wrapped dates in the basket.
4. Place the air fryer basket onto the baking pan.
5. Slide into Rack Position 2, select Air Fry, set Time to 6 minutes, or wait until the bacon is crispy.
6. Remove the dates and allow them to cool on a wire rack for 5 minutes before serving.

Nutrition: Calories: 246 Protein: 14.4g Fiber: 0.6 g Net Carbohydrates: 2.0 g Fat: 17.9 g Sodium: 625 Mg Carbohydrates: 2.6 g

CPSIA information can be obtained
at www.ICGtesting.com
Printed in the USA
BVHW062309160621
609642BV00004B/1002